HOW I LOSE 20 POUNDS IN 30DAYS

(WEIGHT LOSS IS VERY EASY & POSSIBLE)

Introduction:

The Reason everybody needs to use the magic of my weight loss system is that I have used it myself, and it works. I assure you that a little trial will convince you.

Question

For this book to better serve you, ask yourself this

question, why do I need to lose weight?

According to National Heart, Lung and Blood Institute, these are the risks of overweight and obesity.

Being overweight or obese isn't cosmetic problem. These conditions greatly raise our risk for other problems.

1. Being fat or obese will lead you to coronary heart disease (CHD). As our body mass rises, so does your risk for coronary disease (CHD).

CHD according to the NIH institute is a condition in which a waxy substance called plague (plak) builds up inside the coronary arteries. These arteries supply oxygen-rich blood to our heart.

Plague can narrow or block the coronary arteries and reduce blood flow to the heart muscle. This can cause angina or heart disease (angina is chest pain or discomfort). Please contact your physician if you feel of this discomfort.

2. Our chances of having a high blood pressure are greater if you're overweight or obese.

3. Being overweight or obese can lead to stroke. This means that when plague buildup in our arteries because of being overweight or obese. Eventually, an area of plague can rupture, causing a blood clot to form.

If the clot is close to your brain, it blocks the flow of blood and oxygen to our brain and cause a stroke.

4. Being overweight or obese raises your risk for colon, breast, endometrial, and gallbladder cancers.

Summary:

I would want you to think about those 4 major reason above why one should have the consciousness to deal with this problem of obesity. I'm sure as of now you may have other reasons why you need to get rid of any fat in your body. Friend, this book is for you. Tell yourself it is possible to lose weight, if Emmanuel can make it this far, you can! Know today that the choice is yours, and that you are the captain of your ship and the master of your fate. Therefore, get up now and challenge yourself.

CHAPTER 1

THE MIND

My name is Emmanuel, I was weighing 218 pounds, and I had a very big protruding belly. For two years I went to the gym to rid of the fat in my body and in my belly but all was waste of time, every person who had access to me by any means will always ask me, 'when will you give birth to a child'? For years I have not taken this question serious, I always accept it as a good joke, and played over it by rubbing my stomach as a sign of acceptance. In my head, I always believe that the rich are those who has the big belly as a symbol of being wealthy, but all this were lies. Bill Gate, late Steve Job, Warren Buffett, Jack Ma, and many others have no pot belly.

One faithful day I then decided to take a complete look at myself, my age and the opinion of others. Today I have discovered the secret which some people do not want you to know about weight loss. It is simple and easy, it cost less, and very effective way to get rid of any quantity of weight you want to from your body. Truly speaking coaches who knows this secret makes turns of money from celebrities and the famous. I encourage you to read through this book and do what you find well in it because the answer is in the doing. Note, my weight loss success started from the mind, and what I needed was to change my mindset, believing that I can make a change to my body.

My mind became my center of focus because this is where all the thinking for solution will be resolved. The mind is where I will have all the useful questions and answers. Also in in my mind I need to know that I am the captain of my soul, and the master of my fate (William Ernest Henly). I remembered that Napoleon Hill said in his book Think & Grow Rich that, "whatever the mind of a man will conceive and believe, the mind can achieve." So I **conceived and believed** that it is possible for me to lose weight and live long on earth.

As of today I weigh 174 pounds, this is the journey of good health I started one day on my mind and then work on it through the power of imagination, which visualized who I really wanted to be and saw it real in the window of my mind. Today, I look young, sweet, and handsome. I can assure you that when you follow through this book your life and body will be transformed permanently for good.

I am about to reveal to you my simple secret, and this is what people do not want you to know.

According to Earl Nightingale in his book, The Strangest Secret, he said that **"we become**

what we think about," he went further to elaborate that throughout history, philosophers, prophets and great men of wisdom have disagreed with one another on many different things but on the point of we becoming what we think about they are in complete unanimously agreed. Therefore, the key to success and failure in any thing is this: **"we become what we think about."**

Earl Nightingale Mind Theory

He compared the human mind to a farmer's land. **As Ye Sow, So Shall You Reap**

He said I quote, "The human mind is much like a farmer's land. Suppose a farmer has some land. And it is good fertile land. The land gives the farmer a choice. He may plant in that land whatever he chooses. The land doesn't care what is planted. It's up to the farmer to make the decisions.

Nightingale asked me to remember that we are comparing the human mind to the farmer's land because, the mind, like the land, doesn't care what you plant.

Let's say that the farmer has two seeds in his hand- one a seed of corn, the other is nightshade, a deadly poison. He digs two little holes in the earth and he plants both seeds, one corn, the other nightshade.

He covers up the holes, waters, and take care of the land. The question now is, what do you think will happen? Invariably, the land will return what is planted. As it is written in the Bible, **"As ye sow, so shall ye reap."**

Remember, the land doesn't care.

It will return poison in just as wonderful abundance as it will corn. So up come the two plants- one corn, one poison.

According to Nightingale, the human mind is far more fertile, far more incredible and mysterious than the land, but it works the same way. It does not care what we plant whether it is success or failure. A concrete, worthwhile goal or confusion, misunderstanding, fear, anxiety, and so on. But what we plant it must return to us.

The human mind is the last great unexplored continent on earth. It contains riches beyond our wildest dreams. It will return anything we want to plant.

So you may say, if that is true, why don't people use their minds more? According to Earl Nightingale he said that, the problem is that our mind comes as a standard equipment at birth. It's free.

And things that are given to us for nothing, we as human place little value on. Things that we pay money for, we value.

He went further to elaborate that the paradox is that exactly the reverse is true. Everything that's really worthwhile in life came to us free: our minds, our souls, our bodies, our hopes, our dreams, our ambitions, our intelligence, our love of family and children and friends and country. All these priceless possessions are free.

According to Nightingale he went further to emphasized that things that cost us money are very cheap and can be replaced at any time. A good man can be completely wiped out and make another fortune. He can do that several times. Even if our home burns down, we can rebuild it. But the things we got for nothing, we can never replace.

Therefore, the human mind is not used because we take it for granted. It can do any kind of job assign to it, but generally speaking, we use it for little jobs instead of big important ones.

Then the major step to be taken is the decision you make now.

What is it you want?

I guess you want to lose weight and have a healthy body.

Therefore, plant this goal in your mind which may be the most important decision you'll ever make in your entire life.

This question, what is it do I want? Helped me to achieve my goal.

Conclusion:

In conclusion all you have to do is plant that seed in your mind, care for it, work steadily towards your goal, and it will become reality.

Earl Nightingale Counseling:

These things we bring on ourselves through our habitual way of thinking. Every one of us is sum total of our own thoughts.

We are where we are because that is exactly where we really want or feel we deserve to be- whether we'll admit that or not.

Therefore, each of us must live off the fruit of our thoughts in the future, because what you think today and tomorrow, next month and next year will mold your life and determine your future. Know you are guided by your mind.

Weight loss important tips:

- To be successful in selling our way to the good life, we must be willing to pay the price.
- We must be willing to understand emotionally as well as intellectually that we literally become what we think about, that we must control our thoughts if we are to control our lives.
- Realize that our limitation is self-imposed, and the opportunities for you

today are enormous beyond belief.

- Use all your courage to force yourself to think positively on our own problem.
- Set a definite goal and clearly defined goal for yourself
- Let your marvelous mind think about your goal from all possible angles
- Let your imagination speculate freely upon many different possible solutions

- Refuse to believe that there are any circumstances sufficiently strong to defeat you in the accomplishment of your purpose.

Six Steps That Will Help You Realize Success by Dr. David Harold Fink who is an outstanding psychiatrist.

1. Set yourself a definite goal
2. Quit running yourself down

3. Stop thinking of all the reasons why you cannot be successful and instead think of all the reasons why you can

4. Trace your attitudes back through your childhood and discover where you first got the idea that you could not be successful if that is the way you've been thinking.

5. Change the image o have of yourself by writing out description

of the person you would like to be.

6. Act the part of the successful person you have decided to become.

CHAPTER 11

Discipline

The greatest challenge in losing weight is discipline. I discipline myself from eating junk foods especially Chinese food, Macdonald's food, fatty foods like red meat of any kind. I avoid sugar and salt foods and drinks, but rather chose to eat healthy foods such as vegetables, homemade foods and much of protein building foods. Friends I love chicken and beans. Below are some of my healthy foods.

Healthy Foods

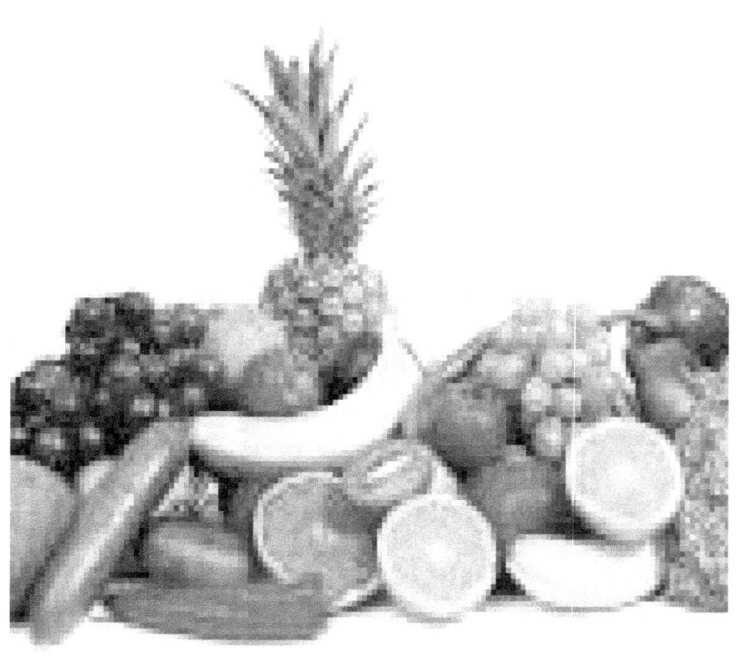

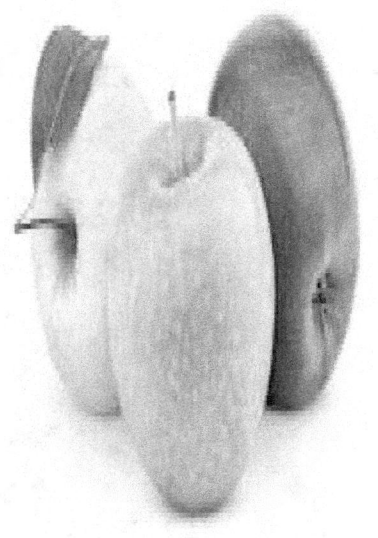

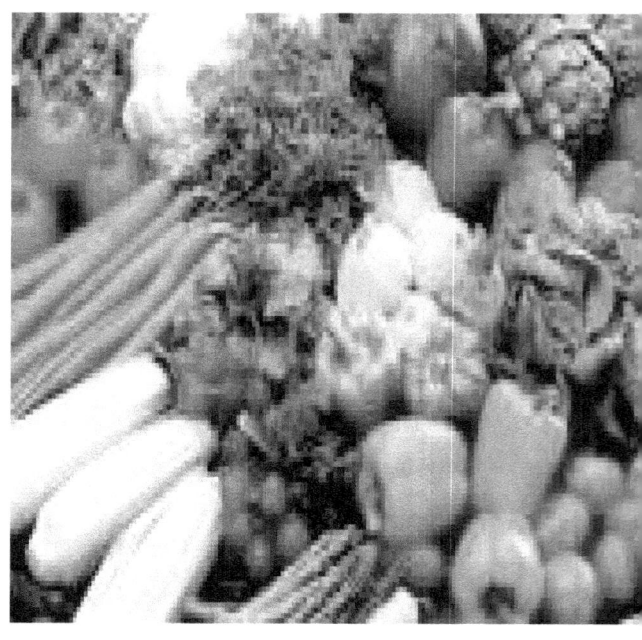

For the first two weeks I ate a lot of fruits, vegetables, drink lots of water and also try to sleep well.

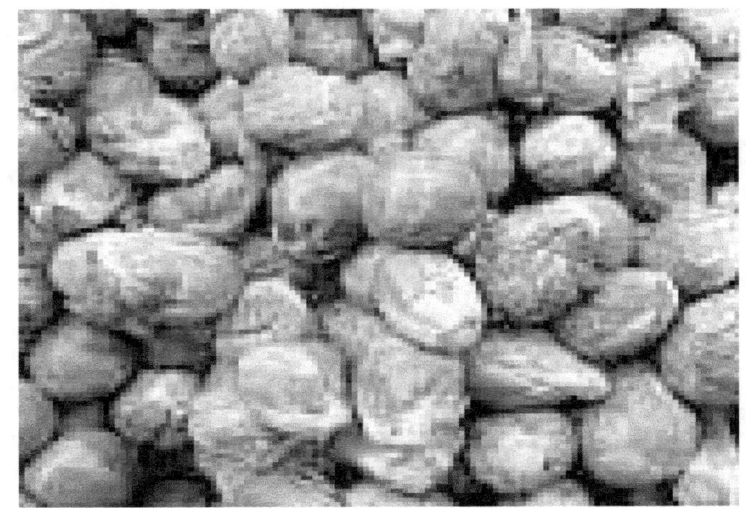

Brussels sprouts

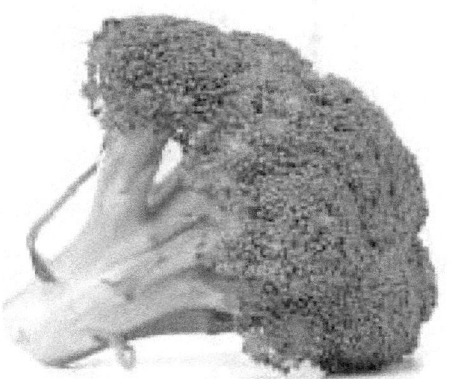

Broccoli

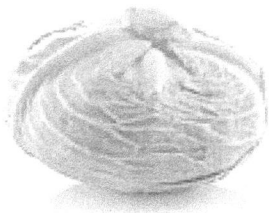

Cabbage

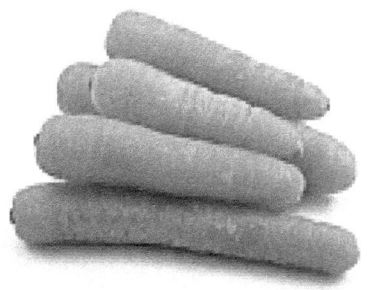

Carrot

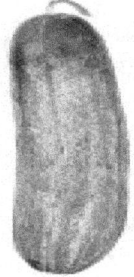

Cucumber

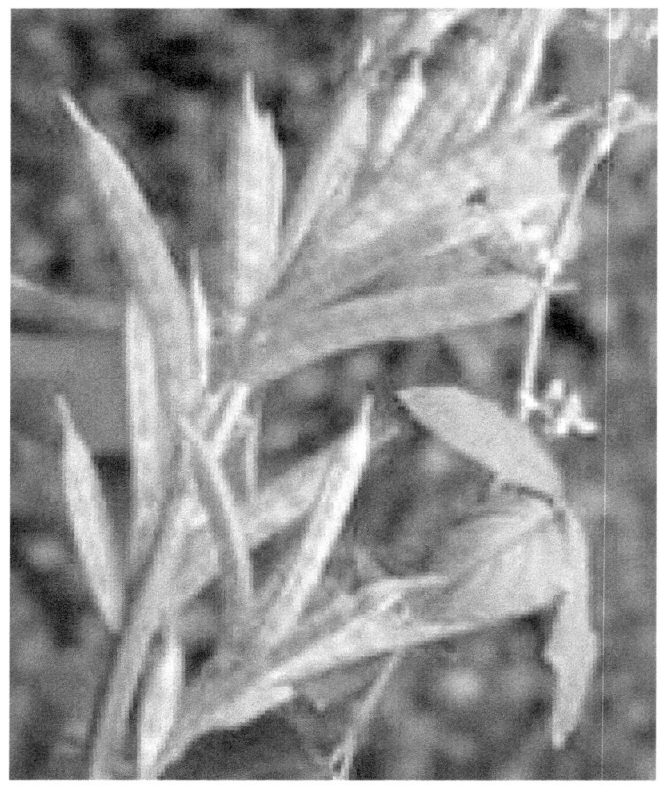

Cluster beans

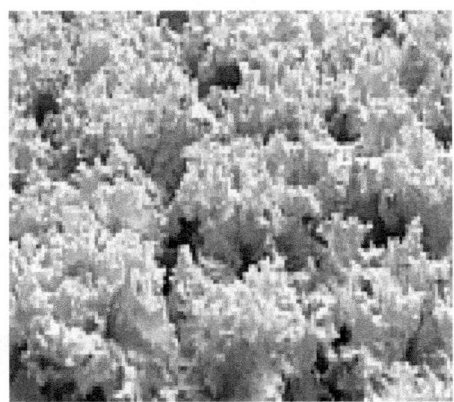

Lettuce

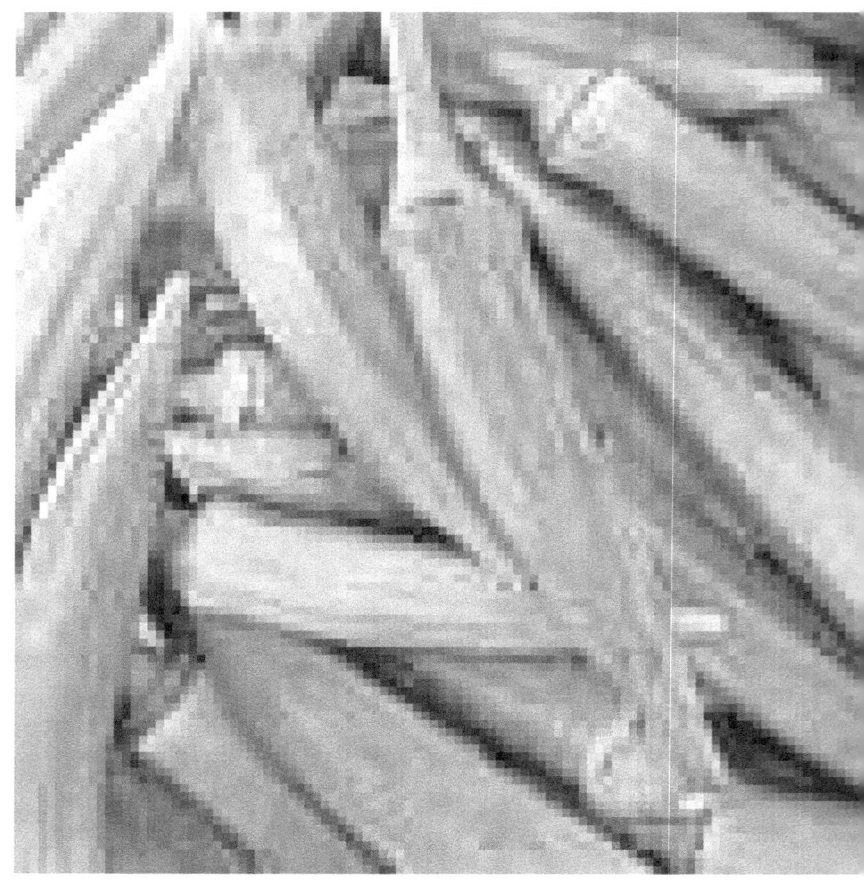

Okra

- For protein, I eat a lot of cooked beans with no salt

- Fish
- Yogurt

Things I keep watch daily.

- I eat little per meal
- I drink much water per meal
- For two weeks I use waist band while eating per meal and stay on it for about 6 to 8hours as desired (waist band helps me not to eat much and controls the belly fat). You can buy waist band at Amazon.com for less than $20.00)

- I eat much fruit per meal (such as blue berry, peas, oranges, banana etc.)
- I eat a lot of nuts
- And finally I use my common sense to decide what food is good for my body by searching through the internet.

Chapter 111

Fasting

Fasting is another way I used to cleanse my system both spiritually and physically. Through fasting everything patterning to the flesh such as the craving for junk foods will be brought under the subjection to God and myself. During this period, I am surrendering all my will to God, presenting my request to him that I am ready to lose weight or achieve the goals set before me, and that for His help I am confidence to achieve it.

It worked for me, so it will also work for you.

The Holy Bible said that when you fast.

1. Your light will break forth as morning.
2. Your health shall spring forth speedily.
3. Your light shall rise in obscurity.

- Note, I fast once a week by my own choice.

A Strong Word of encouragement from Napoleon Hill from Think & Grow Rich.

"If you think you are beaten, you are,

If you think you dare not, you don't.

If you like to win, but you think you can't. It is almost certain you won't

"If you think you'll lose, you're lost,

For out in the world we find,

Success begins with a fellow's will

It's all in the state of mind.

"If you think you outclassed, you are,

You've got to think high to rise,

You've got be sure of yourself before

You can ever win a prize.

"Life's battles don't always go

To the stronger or faster man,

But soon or late the man who wins

Is the man who thinks he can

Chapter iv

Exercise

With my principle you need just a little exercise each day. Just 10 minutes of exercise will give you the strength that will carry you through the day. Read this weight loss magic book, do what it tells you to do for 30 days. I am assuring you that you will testify that it works and that you have lost 20 pounds. Then, if you want to lose more continue to repeat what you've known for the magic is in obedience and practice.

You don't need to go to the gym any more for weight loss, follow my method which is what I did, and after that you can go to the gym for strength and continual fitness. My system comes first, walk a little distance each day, play music and dance at home, then wait and see the result yourself.

I wish you good luck in this journey of good health.

Feel free to write me @ emmanuellegend@yahoo.com or call me @ (267)423 5695 or book me @ www.johncmaxwellgroup.com /emmanueludoeyo

Remember: "Whatever the mind of a man can conceive and believe, it can achieve." Napoleon Hill

"All things are possible to them that believes." Bible

"As a man thinks in his heart so is he." Bible

30 Day Action Ideas for Putting My Weight Loss Secret to Work for You

I've explained the magic of my weight loss secret, and how it works. Now I'd like to explain how you can prove to yourself the enormous returns possible in your own life by putting the secret to a practical test.

I want you to make a practice test that will last 30 days. If you give it a good try, though it is not easy, but it will completely change your life for better.

Sir Isaac Newton said, "For every action, there is an equal and opposite reaction." This means we can achieve nothing without paying some sort of price.

Therefore, for this 30 days be aware of the following;

1. Understand intellectually and emotionally that you must control your thoughts because literally you become what you think about.

2. Cut away all fetters from your mind knowing that

your limitations are self-imposed.

3. Use your courage to force yourself to think positively on your own problem, and also refuse to believe that there are any circumstances sufficiently strong to defeat you in the accomplishment of your purpose.

4. Finally, write down on a card how weight you want to loss. Carry the card with you so that you look at it several times a day. Think of your goals in a

cheerful, relaxed, positive way each morning when you get up, and praise yourself for each accomplishment.

Simple Exercises for the Body

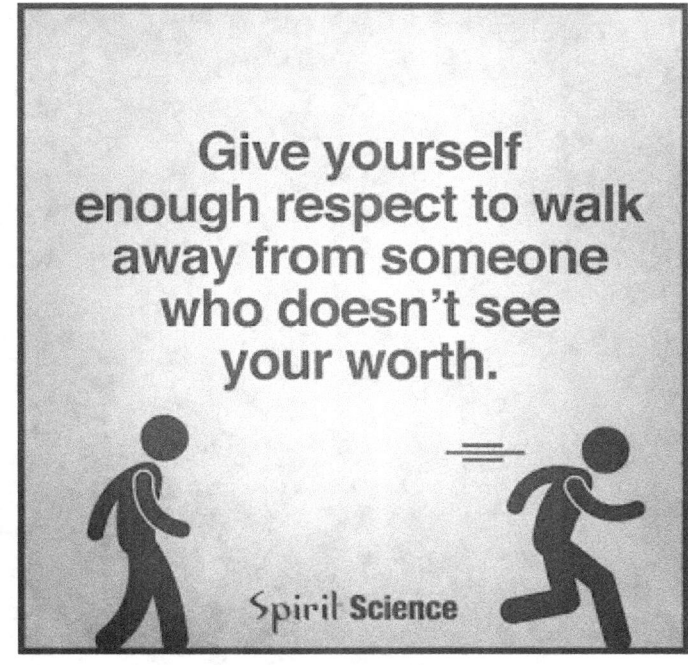

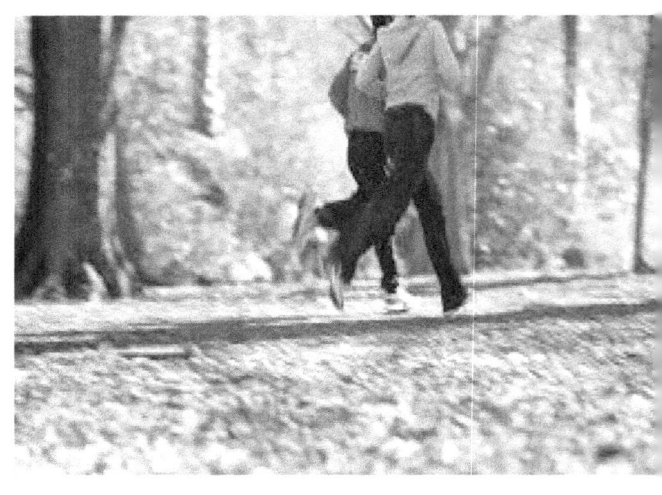

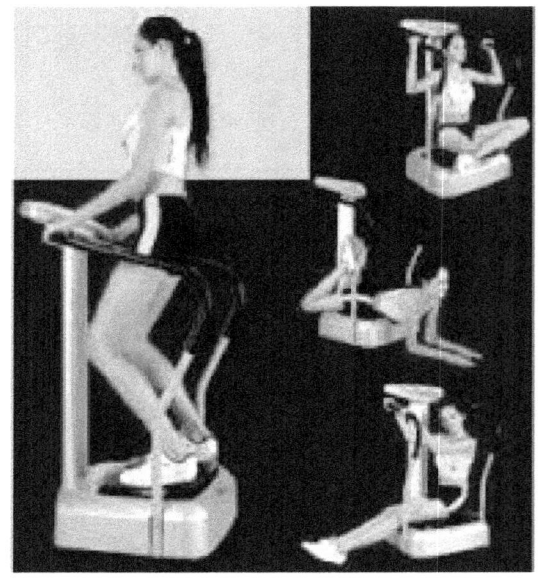

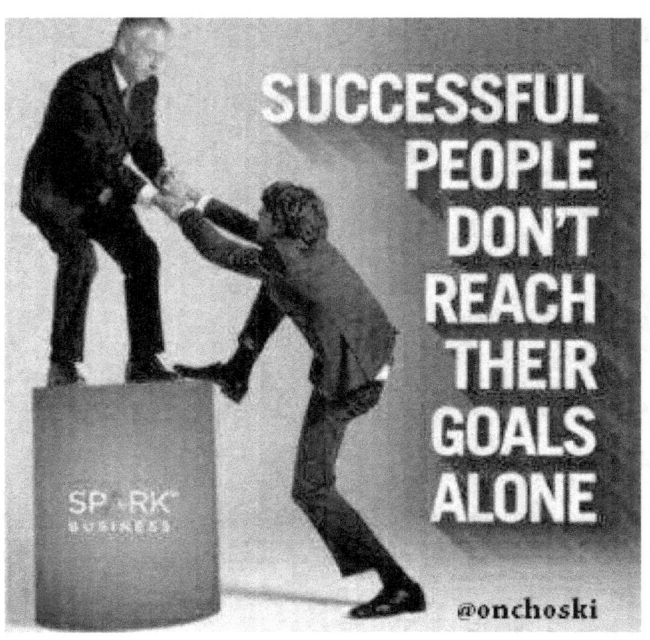

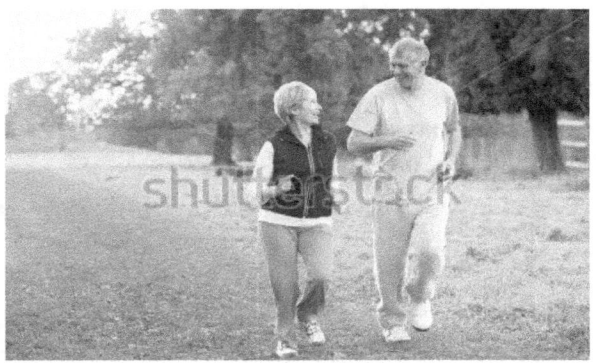

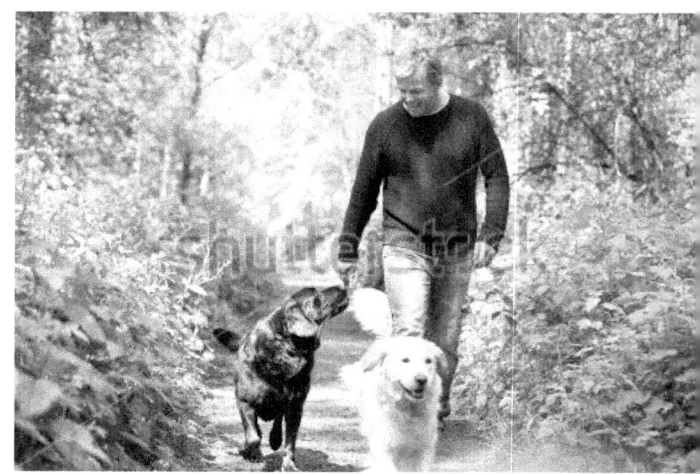

www.shutterstock.com · 270164993

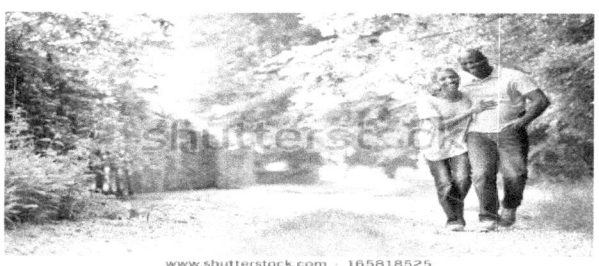

www.shutterstock.com · 165818525

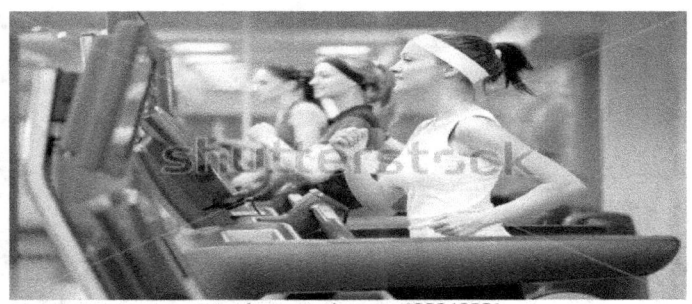

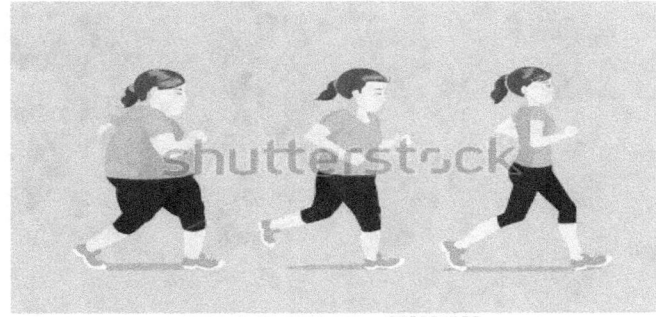

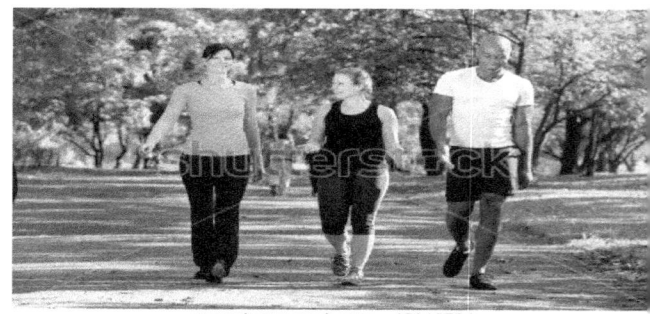

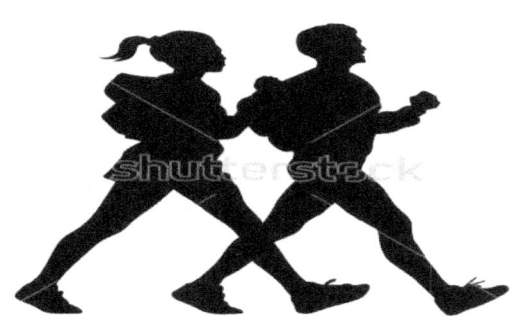

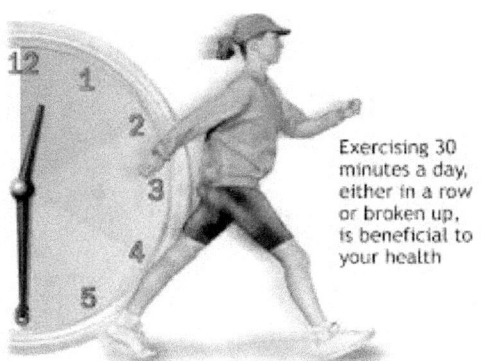

Exercising 30 minutes a day, either in a row or broken up, is beneficial to your health